UTI Mastery:

The Future of Urinary Tract Health

By

Richard L. Magee

The writers and publishers do not promote or advocate any particular medical treatments, drugs, or procedures. Any choices on healthcare or medical treatments should be made in consultation with healthcare specialists.

This book may provide generic descriptions of medical disorders, their causes, and possible remedies. It is crucial to remember that individual instances may differ, and each person's medical demands and circumstances are unique. Consequently, the material in this book should be treated as a general reference rather than a replacement for customized medical advice.

The writers and publishers disclaim all responsibility for any loss, injury, or damage caused as a consequence of the information in this book or any reliance on it. The writers and publishers are not responsible for the content of any websites or resources that may be referenced or linked in this book.

Readers should always seek the counsel of a certified healthcare practitioner before making any choices about their health and well-being.

Table of Contents

INTRODUCTION

In the huge range of health issues that impact millions of people worldwide, few ailments are as ubiquitous, but frequently disregarded, as urinary tract infections (UTIs). While these illnesses may be ubiquitous, their influence on people's lives and well-being is not to be ignored. A UTI may vary from a slight nuisance to a cause of severe discomfort, pain, and even major health issues.

"UTI Mastery: The Future of Urinary Tract Health " is a book that tries to shed light on this often misunderstood medical disease. In the pages that follow, we will start on a voyage of discovery, digging into the complexity of UTIs, their origins, symptoms, prevention, and therapies. Our voyage will take us through the structure of the urinary system, the numerous forms of UTIs, the ways they impact different populations, and the current breakthroughs in detection and treatment.

This book is aimed to serve as a beneficial resource for anyone seeking information and empowerment in controlling their urinary health. It is for the caregivers who seek to provide compassionate assistance and for the healthcare professionals devoted to giving the finest care to their patients. As we explore the realm of UTIs, we will reveal not only the scientific and medical aspects but also the human and emotional sides of these diseases.

Our objective is to provide you with the information and resources to navigate the world of UTIs with confidence, whether you are attempting to avoid them, battling to manage their recurrence, or hoping to assist a loved one on their road to recovery. "Understanding UTIs" encourages you to go on an informative examination of a ubiquitous, but sometimes underestimated, medical condition, presenting insights that will empower you to take care of your urinary health and general well-being.

CHAPTER ONE

UNDERSTANDING UTIs

How Our Urinary System Works

The urinary system, also known as the renal system, is a complicated and crucial element of the human body responsible for maintaining internal balance and general health. Its tasks are diverse, spanning the filtering of waste and surplus chemicals from the circulation to generate urine, management of the composition and volume of blood, maintenance of electrolyte balance, and support of important processes such as blood pressure regulation. To comprehend the urinary system, let's investigate its workings in further depth:

1. Kidneys: The Filtration Powerhouse

The process originates in the kidneys, two extraordinary, bean-shaped organs situated below the ribcage on each side of the spine. These organs serve a key role in maintaining internal balance. Each kidney includes over a million small filtering units called nephrons, responsible for the important process of blood filtration.

2. Filtration: The Nephron's Role

Blood reaches the nephrons by a network of small arteries, notably the afferent arterioles. Within the nephrons, blood undergoes a basic transformation: it is separated into two components - the filtrate and the remaining blood. The filtrate includes waste products including urea, creatinine, and excessive salts, together with important chemicals that need reabsorption.

3. Formation of Urine: A Multistep Process

The transition of filtrate into urine comprises several important stages:

- **Reabsorption:** As the filtrate travels the complicated labyrinth of the nephron, several important chemicals, including water, glucose, and electrolytes, are selectively reabsorbed from the filtrate back into the circulation. This mechanism ensures that important compounds are retained, avoiding their loss in the urine.

- **Concentration:** Following reabsorption, the leftover filtrate, now known as urine, continues its trip along the renal tubules. These tubules are crucial in further concentrating the urine, mostly by removing more water and concentrating waste materials.

4. Collection: The Renal Pelvis

The now concentrated urine is collected in the renal pelvis, a funnel-shaped structure situated inside each kidney. This represents the initial stage in the travel of urine from the kidneys to the outside of the body.

5. Ureters: Transporting Urine

Urine departs the kidneys via the ureters, small tubes that carry it to the urinary bladder. Peristaltic contractions in the ureters assist in driving urine down the route, ensuring that it reaches the bladder for storage.

6. Bladder: The Urine Reservoir

The urinary bladder is a muscular sac that works as a storage reservoir for urine. It has the extraordinary capacity to expand and compress, accommodating various quantities of urine. Sensory neurons inside the bladder notify the brain when it is full, giving rise to the conscious sense of wanting to urinate.

7. Voiding: The Act of Urination

When the bladder exceeds its capacity, messages are conveyed to the brain, producing the conscious knowledge of the urge to pee. At this point, a sphincter muscle at the base of the bladder relaxes, while the bladder's muscular wall contracts, discharging urine down the urethra. 8. Urethra: The Exit Path

The urethra is the last component of the urinary system. It operates as the route via which urine escapes the body. In men, the urethra has a dual duty, supporting both the urine and reproductive systems. In females, it mainly acts as a route for the outflow of urine.

This thorough process of filtration, reabsorption, concentration, and excretion is vital to the body's general health and well-being. The urinary system's unceasing functioning guarantees the elimination of metabolic waste products, maintenance of water and electrolyte balance, and the retention of essential compounds in the circulation. Furthermore, the urinary system plays a crucial function in the control of blood pressure, red blood cell synthesis, and the maintenance of acid-base balance in the body. Understanding the complexity of the urinary system provides insight into its important role in preserving the body's internal homeostasis.

Different Types of UTIs

1. Cystitis (Bladder Infection)

Cystitis is the most prevalent kind of UTI and mostly affects the bladder. It is commonly referred to as a "lower UTI." Cystitis often comes from germs, most frequently Escherichia coli (E. coli), invading the bladder. Symptoms of cystitis include frequent urination, a strong need to pee, a burning feeling during urination, murky or bloody urine, and pain or pressure in the lower abdomen. While cystitis is often not as serious as kidney infections, it may be painful and irritating.

2. Pyelonephritis (Kidney Infection):

Pyelonephritis is a more severe UTI that affects the kidneys. It is commonly referred to as an "upper UTI." This syndrome may occur from untreated or repeated bladder infections that ascend to the kidneys. Symptoms of pyelonephritis include high fever, chills, back or side discomfort (flank pain), nausea, and vomiting. It needs quick medical care and may be connected with more serious problems.

3. Urethritis:

Urethritis is a UTI that affects the urethra, the tube linking the bladder to the exterior of the body. It may be caused by both bacterial and non-bacterial causes, including sexually transmitted infections (STIs) like chlamydia and gonorrhea. Symptoms of urethritis include discomfort or a burning feeling during urination, increased urine frequency, and discharge from the urethra. It is more frequent in women, although males may also have urethritis.

4. Prostatitis (Prostate Infection):

Prostatitis is an infection or inflammation of the prostate gland, a walnut-sized gland found directly below the bladder in males. Prostatitis may be either acute or chronic. Symptoms may include discomfort in the lower abdomen, lower back, or perineum, uncomfortable urination, fever, or chills. Prostatitis may be caused by bacterial or non-bacterial causes. It might be tough to identify and treat.

5. Asymptomatic Bacteriuria:

Asymptomatic bacteriuria refers to the presence of bacteria in the urine without presenting any symptoms. It is typically discovered inadvertently during regular urine testing and may not need treatment, particularly in some groups, including pregnant women. However, in rare circumstances, it may be managed to avoid problems.

6. Recurrent UTIs:

Some patients encounter numerous UTIs over time, typically with identical symptoms. Recurrent UTIs may affect any component of the urinary system. In such circumstances, healthcare experts may propose additional examination to uncover underlying reasons, contributing variables, and preventive actions to limit the recurrence of UTIs.

7. Complicated UTIs:

Complicated UTIs are those that occur in persons with characteristics that make the infection more complex to treat. Complications might include urinary tract anomalies, blockages, kidney stones, pregnancy, diabetes, compromised immune systems, or catheter usage. Treatment of severe UTIs sometimes involves a more complete examination and may entail a longer course of antibiotics.

What Causes UTIs

1. **Bacterial Invasion:** The most prevalent cause of UTIs is the entrance of bacteria into the urinary system. Among the key causes is Escherichia coli (E.coli), a bacteria that normally inhabits the gastrointestinal system. When these bacteria migrate from the rectal region to the urethra, they may climb into the urinary system and cause illness.

2. **Sexual Activity:** Sexual intercourse may transfer germs into the urethra, increasing the risk of UTIs, especially in women. This illness is commonly referred to as "honeymoon cystitis."

3. **Urinary Tract Obstructions:** Conditions that block or interfere with the natural flow of urine might heighten the risk of UTIs. Common blockages include kidney stones, urinary tract abnormalities, and disorders that induce urine retention.

4. **Anatomical features:** Some persons have anatomical features that may predispose them to UTIs. For example,

women often have shorter urethras than males, making it
simpler for germs to enter the bladder.

5. **Catheter Use:** Urinary catheters, widely utilized in hospital
settings, may introduce germs into the urinary system,
raising the probability of catheter-associated UTIs.

6. **Weakened Immune System:** A damaged immune system,
arising from illnesses like diabetes, HIV/AIDS, or the use
of immunosuppressive medicines, may limit the body's
capacity to fight off infections, including UTIs.

7. **Urinary Retention:** Incomplete emptying of the bladder
may produce an environment conducive to bacterial
development and raise the risk of infection. Conditions
include an enlarged prostate in males or neurological
problems that may contribute to urine retention.

8. **Postmenopausal Changes:** In postmenopausal women,
hormonal changes may result in numerous physiological
modifications in the urinary system, such as a thinner and
less protective vaginal lining, rendering them more prone to
UTIs.

9. **Pregnancy:** During pregnancy, hormonal changes may contribute to urinary stasis (restricted urine flow), increasing the risk of UTIs. Pregnant women should be more attentive to UTI prevention and control.

10. **Childhood UTIs:** In children, UTIs may be linked with congenital urinary tract anomalies, vesicoureteral reflux (the backward flow of urine from the bladder into the ureters), or other structural difficulties.

11. **Sexually Transmitted diseases (STIs):** Certain sexually transmitted diseases (STIs), such as chlamydia and gonorrhea, may lead to urethritis (inflammation of the urethra). This inflammation might render the urinary system more vulnerable to UTIs.

12. **Previous UTIs:** Individuals who have suffered UTIs in the past may be at an elevated risk of repeat infections. Addressing possible underlying issues and taking preventive actions might help lessen the chance of recurrence.

13. **Use of Spermicides and Diaphragms:** Some contraceptive techniques, such as spermicides and

diaphragms, might affect the vaginal flora and pH, possibly making it easier for bacteria to cause UTIs.

Understanding the numerous causes and risk factors connected with UTIs is crucial for people to take proactive actions to avoid these infections.

CHAPTER TWO

RECOGNIZING UTIS

Signs and Symptoms of UTIs

1. Cystitis (Bladder Infection):

- **Frequent Urination:** Individuals with cystitis typically feel the urge to pee more often than normal. This increased frequency may occur even when there is very little pee in the bladder.

- **Need:** Along with frequent urination, there's a sensation of the need to pee, making it difficult to postpone going to the toilet.

- **Dysuria (Painful urinating):** A burning, stinging, or pain during urinating is a defining symptom of cystitis.

- **Hematuria:** Cystitis may lead to the presence of blood in the urine, making it look pink, red, or murky.

- **Foul-Smelling Urine:** Urine may take on an unpleasant odor owing to the illness.

-

- **Lower Abdominal Discomfort:** Some people may suffer mild to moderate discomfort or pressure in the lower abdomen or pelvic area.
- **General Malaise:** Feeling generally sick, weary, or having a low-grade fever may accompany cystitis.

2. Pyelonephritis (Kidney Infection):

- High temperature with Chills: Individuals with pyelonephritis commonly experience a high temperature, which may be accompanied by shaking and chills.
- **Flank Pain:** The pain in pyelonephritis is generally centered in the lower back, below the ribs, and may be intense and constant.
- **Nausea and Vomiting:** In addition to the pain and fever, nausea and vomiting are frequent symptoms of kidney infections.
- **Dysuria:** Painful urination may also be a symptom of pyelonephritis.

- **Urgent desire to pee:** Individuals may have an urgent desire to pee, even if they have already emptied their bladder.
- **Cloudy, Bloody, or Foul-Smelling Urine:** Similar to cystitis, pyelonephritis may result in changes in urine appearance and odor.

3. Urethritis:

- **Pain or Burning Sensation During Urination:** Urethritis mainly presents as pain or a burning sensation while passing urine.
- **Increased Frequency of Urination:** Individuals with urethritis may urinate more often than normal.
- **Urethral Discharge:** Some may notice a discharge from the urethra, which might vary in color and consistency.
- **Mild Lower abdomen Pain:** Discomfort in the lower abdomen region is another possible sign.

4. Prostatitis (Prostate Infection):

- **Lower Abdominal or Pelvic Pain:** Pain or discomfort is commonly felt in the lower abdomen, lower back, perineum (the region between the genitals and anus), or rectum.

- **Painful or Burning Urination**: Similar to other UTIs, painful urination is a typical symptom.

- **Urgent or Frequent Urination:** A frequent desire to pee, even with small urine output, might develop.

- **Systemic Symptoms:** Fever and chills may be present, especially in acute prostatitis.

- **Urinary Retention:** In rare circumstances, prostatitis may cause difficulties in beginning or sustaining urination.

5. Asymptomatic Bacteriuria:

- In situations of asymptomatic bacteriuria, there are no apparent signs. The presence of germs in the urine is determined by laboratory testing during regular check-ups or screenings.

6. Recurrent UTIs:

For persons with recurrent UTIs, the symptoms tend to be identical to those mentioned above. However, the frequency of infections may lead to a pattern of recurring bouts of bladder pain, which may vary in degree.

It's crucial to realize that the presentation of UTI symptoms may vary greatly, and some patients, particularly the elderly, may suffer unusual or more mild symptoms, such as disorientation, agitation, or inexplicable falls.

When to See a Doctor

Seeing a doctor for a urinary tract infection (UTI) is vital to ensure accurate diagnosis and treatment. While some mild UTIs may clear on their own, untreated or severe UTIs may develop complications, such as kidney infections, which can be more problematic and need more thorough treatment. Here are some tips on when to consult a doctor for a UTI:

1. **Symptoms of a UTI:** If you suffer classic UTI symptoms, such as a frequent, urgent need to pee, burning during urination, and murky, bloody, or strong-smelling urine, it's important to consult a doctor soon. Other symptoms, such as flank discomfort, fever, and vomiting (showing a

probable kidney infection), should also lead you to seek medical assistance.

2. **Recurrent UTIs:** If you've had many UTIs in the past, particularly within a short period, it's crucial to contact a healthcare practitioner. They may assist in discovering any underlying causes or contributing factors and offer preventive methods.

3. **Asymptomatic Bacteriuria:** If you are pregnant, old, or have certain medical concerns, your healthcare practitioner may test your urine at regular check-ups. whether asymptomatic bacteriuria is identified, your doctor will assess whether treatment is essential to avoid consequences.

4. **Children**: If a youngster suffers from UTI symptoms, it's necessary to visit a physician. UTIs in children might occasionally be accompanied by underlying disorders that require additional assessment.

5. **Elderly Individuals:** In the elderly, UTI symptoms may be unusual, and disorientation or agitation might be evidence of an underlying infection. Family members and caregivers

should be watchful and see a healthcare physician if they suspect a UTI.

6. **Pain or Discomfort Persists:** If you feel chronic discomfort or pain in the lower abdomen, lower back, or pelvic region, particularly when accompanied by urinary symptoms, it's crucial to seek medical help.

7. **Recurrent urine difficulties:** If you experience chronic urine difficulties, such as frequent urination, urgency, or incontinence, that worsen or are accompanied by discomfort, visit a healthcare practitioner. These symptoms may be connected to a UTI or an underlying ailment.

8. **Catheter Use:** Individuals with urinary catheters are at greater risk of UTIs. If you suffer symptoms of a UTI, especially if you have a catheter, it's crucial to visit a healthcare specialist.

9. **Severe Symptoms:** If you feel severe pain, high fever, chills, or vomiting, it may suggest a more serious illness, such as pyelonephritis (a kidney infection), and needs emergency medical treatment.

10. **Persistent or Recurrent Infections:** If UTIs reoccur often or if symptoms continue or worsen after taking antibiotics, visit your healthcare practitioner. This may suggest antibiotic resistance or an underlying problem that requires additional examination.

It's crucial not to procrastinate obtaining medical assistance for a UTI. Early diagnosis and treatment may help ease symptoms, clear the infection, and avoid consequences.

How Doctors Diagnose UTIs

Diagnosing a urinary tract infection (UTI) often includes a mix of medical history, physical examination, and laboratory investigations. The technique may vary significantly based on the healthcare provider's approach, however below is a broad outline of how UTIs are diagnosed:

1. Medical History:

- Your healthcare professional will begin by questioning you about your symptoms, including the type and length of your urine problems. They will question any discomfort, pain, fever, chills, and changes in the color or smell of your urine.

2. Physical Examination:

- A physical examination may be undertaken, particularly if you have more severe or unusual symptoms. The examination may involve evaluating for discomfort in the lower abdomen or back and screening for indicators of disease, such as fever or dehydration.

3. Urine Sample:

- The most frequent diagnostic test for a UTI is a urine sample. You will be required to give a clean-catch urine sample, which entails the following steps:

  ➢ Wash your hands thoroughly.

  ➢ Clean the genital region with a specific towelette or soap and water.

  ➢ Begin peeing into the toilet, then collect a "midstream" sample of urine in a sterile container given by your healthcare professional.

  ➢ Finish urinating into the toilet.

4. Urine Culture:

- In many circumstances, a urine sample will be submitted to a laboratory for a urine culture. This test identifies the exact bacteria causing the illness and helps identify which drugs will be most successful in treating the condition. It takes a day or two to acquire the results from a urine culture.

5. Urine Dipstick Test:

- A urine dipstick test may offer immediate findings by detecting particular chemicals in the urine, such as white blood cells (indicating infection), nitrites (frequently caused by bacteria), and blood. While a positive result signals a suspected UTI, a urine culture is often required for confirmation and to identify the exact bacteria.

6. Blood Tests:

- In certain situations, particularly if you have symptoms indicative of a more serious infection (e.g., kidney infection), blood tests may be conducted to monitor kidney function and discover any evidence of systemic infection.

7. Imaging Studies:

- In some instances, such as when UTIs are recurring or accompanied by uncommon symptoms, imaging procedures like ultrasonography, computed tomography (CT), or magnetic resonance imaging (MRI) may be indicated to screen for structural abnormalities in the urinary tract.

8. Cystoscopy:

- A cystoscopy is a technique that includes utilizing a thin, flexible tube with a camera to inspect the interior of the urethra and bladder. It may be indicated if you have recurring UTIs, atypical symptoms, or other concerns regarding the urinary system.

9. Pediatric Evaluation:

- For children with UTI symptoms, a doctor may utilize additional assessment methods, such as kidney ultrasounds, to screen for urinary tract abnormalities.

CHAPTER THREE

PREVENTING UTIs

Simple Ways to Avoid UTIs

Urinary tract infections (UTIs) may be unpleasant and bothersome, but there are numerous easy strategies to lower your chance of acquiring them. Here are some simple and efficient techniques to prevent UTIs:

1. **Stay Hydrated:** Drinking a sufficient quantity of water is vital for having a healthy urinary system. It helps flush out germs and reduces concentrated urine, which may lead to UTIs. Aim for at least 8 cups (64 ounces) of water every day.

2. **Regular urinating:** Don't postpone urinating when you feel the urge. Frequent emptying of the bladder may help clear out any dangerous germs before an illness can develop.

3. **Proper Wiping:** Always wipe from front to back after using the toilet. This limits the movement of germs from

the anal region to the urethra, minimizing the risk of infection.

4. **Urinate After Sex:** After sexual activity, urinate to help flush out any germs that may have entered the urethra during intercourse.

5. **Proper Personal Hygiene:** Maintain proper genital hygiene by keeping the region clean and dry. Avoid using strong soaps, douches, or scented items that might irritate the urethra.

6. **Avoid Irritants:** Refrain from using goods that may irritate the urinary system, such as bubble baths, scented toilet paper, and feminine hygiene sprays.

7. **Cranberry Products:** While studies are inconsistent, some individuals find that cranberry juice or supplements help prevent UTIs by making it more difficult for germs to cling to the urinary system walls.

8. **Breathable Clothing:** Choose breathable, cotton undergarments and avoid tight-fitting pants. Breathable textiles help keep the genital region dry, minimizing excessive bacterial development.

9. **Spermicides and Diaphragms:** If you use spermicides or diaphragms for contraception and encounter recurring UTIs, explore alternate birth control options. These products may affect vaginal flora and pH, making it easier for bacteria to cause UTIs.

10. **Lubricants:** If you use lubricants during sexual activity, pick water-based, unscented choices to avoid the risk of irritation or disturbance of the vaginal flora.

11. **Probiotics:** Some persons take probiotics containing helpful bacteria, since they may assist in maintaining a healthy balance of flora in the urinary system. Consult with a healthcare practitioner for information on utilizing probiotics.

12. **Medical Evaluation:** If you encounter recurring UTIs, underlying medical issues, or anatomical characteristics that make you more prone to UTIs, check with a healthcare practitioner. They might propose extra preventative measures or drugs.

13. **Avoid Holding Urine:** Try to react soon when you sense the urge to pee. Holding in urine may create an environment where germs can grow.

14. **Regular Exercise:** Engaging in regular physical exercise may help overall health and may indirectly promote the health of the urinary tract.

15. **Wipe and Hydrate Properly During Menstruation:** During menstruation, maintain appropriate hygiene by changing sanitary products often and maintaining cleanliness. Proper hydration is also vital.

16. **Post-Menopausal Care:** Postmenopausal women may consider exploring hormone replacement therapy or other alternatives with their healthcare providers to address the increased susceptibility to UTIs linked with hormonal changes.

It's crucial to realize that although these prophylactic steps may help minimize the incidence of UTIs, they may not ensure total immunity. If you have signs of a UTI, such as discomfort during urinating, frequent urination, or changes in urine color or odor, get quick medical assistance. Early diagnosis and treatment may help avoid problems and ease pain.

Eating and Drinking for UTI Prevention

Certain foods and drinks may help your urinary tract health by boosting your immune system and supporting overall well-being. Here are dietary and hydration guidelines for UTI prevention:

1. **Drink Plenty of Water:** Staying well-hydrated is one of the most critical things you can take to avoid UTIs. Adequate water consumption helps dilute urine and wash away pathogens from the urinary system. Aim for at least 8 cups (64 ounces) of water every day, and more if you're physically active or live in a hot region.

2. **Unsweetened Cranberry Juice:** Some research shows that unsweetened cranberry juice may help prevent UTIs. Cranberries include chemicals that make it harder for germs to attach to the urinary tract walls. However, moderation is crucial, since excessive use might lead to sugar intake. Opt for pure cranberry juice or cranberry pills if you like.

3. **Probiotics:** Probiotic-rich foods, such as yogurt with live cultures or fermented foods such as sauerkraut and kimchi, may help maintain a healthy gut microbiota. A healthy gut flora may indirectly improve urinary tract health by generating a stronger immune system.

4. **Vitamin C:** Foods high in vitamin C, such as citrus fruits, strawberries, and kiwi, may help enhance your immune system. Vitamin C acidifies the urine, which might make it more difficult for germs to flourish.

5. **Garlic:** Garlic is recognized for its antibacterial qualities. Incorporating garlic into your meals may help enhance your body's natural defenses against infections, including UTIs.

6. **Berries:** Blueberries, strawberries, and other berries include antioxidants and minerals that may promote general health and may help minimize the incidence of UTIs.

7. **Leafy Greens:** Leafy greens like spinach, kale, and collard greens are filled with vitamins and minerals that boost your immune system.

8. **Whole Grains:** Whole grains, such as brown rice, quinoa, and whole wheat, contain critical nutrients and fiber that may enhance general well-being.

9. **Lean Proteins:** Lean protein sources, such as chicken, turkey, fish, and tofu, contain necessary amino acids that are vital for a robust immune system.

10. **Foods High in Fiber:** A diet high in fiber helps encourage regular bowel movements, minimizing the risk of constipation. Constipation may exert strain on the urinary system, thus raising the risk of UTIs. Include whole grains, veggies, and fruits in your diet to enhance fiber intake.

11. **Limit Sugar and Refined carbs:** Excess sugar and refined carbs may significantly influence gut health and the immune system. Minimize your consumption of sugary snacks, candies, and white bread.

12. **Moderation with Dairy:** Some persons may find that dairy items increase UTI symptoms. If you suspect this, try lowering or eliminating dairy in your diet.

13. **Avoid Excessive Caffeine and Alcohol:** Caffeine and alcohol may serve as diuretics, possibly contributing to dehydration. Moderation is crucial, and ensure you keep appropriately hydrated while ingesting these drinks.

14. **Balanced Diet:** Maintaining a well-balanced diet that includes a range of fruits, vegetables, whole grains, lean meats, and healthy fats may help with general health and a stronger immune system.

UTI Prevention for Special Cases

Preventing urinary tract infections (UTIs) in unusual instances may need more attention and specialized procedures. Here are UTI preventive measures for these distinct scenarios:

UTI Prevention for Children:

1. **Promote Good Hygiene:** Teach youngsters, particularly girls, the necessity of wiping from front to back after using the toilet to avoid the passage of germs from the anal region to the urethra.

2. **Avoid Bubble Baths:** Discourage the use of bubble baths and strong soaps, which may irritate the vaginal region and make it more prone to infections.

3. **Encourage Regular restroom Breaks:** Make sure youngsters take regular restroom breaks to clear their bladders. Holding in urine may provide circumstances for germs to flourish.

4. **Stay Hydrated:** Ensure your youngster drinks enough water to maintain optimum hydration. Teach children the necessity of regular liquid consumption.

5. **Urinate After Swimming:** Encourage urinating after swimming in pools, since the toxins in pool water might lead to UTIs.

6. **Avoid Tight clothes**: Dress children in loose, breathable clothes to avoid friction and encourage appropriate airflow

UTI Prevention for Seniors:

1. **Stay Hydrated:** Seniors generally have diminished feelings of thirst, rendering them prone to dehydration. Encourage regular hydration intake to avoid UTIs.

2. **Prompt Voiding:** Remind elders to react swiftly to the desire to pee. Delaying urinating might raise the risk of UTIs.

3. **Manage Incontinence:** If incontinence is an issue, ensure that elders have access to absorbent items and maintain excellent hygiene to minimize skin irritation and UTIs.

4. **Review drugs:** Some drugs may raise the risk of UTIs. Discuss pharmaceutical side effects and interactions with a healthcare practitioner.

5. **Hormone Replacement treatment:** In postmenopausal women, hormone replacement treatment may help address the increased susceptibility to UTIs linked with hormonal changes. Consult with a healthcare practitioner to explore possible solutions.

6. **Assist with Personal Hygiene:** Assist elders with maintaining excellent personal hygiene, particularly if mobility or cognitive impairments make self-care difficult.

7. **Frequent Medical Check-ups:** Encourage the elderly to attend frequent medical check-ups. Healthcare practitioners

may detect and manage any health issues, including diseases that may lead to UTIs.

8. **Prevent Constipation:** Constipation may put a strain on the urinary system, increasing the risk of UTIs. Encourage elders to maintain a high-fiber diet and be physically active.

9. **Regular Exercise:** Promote physical exercise to preserve general health, particularly the health of the urinary tract.

10. **Correct Catheter Care:** If a senior uses a urinary catheter, ensure that it is well-maintained, and follow correct catheter care recommendations to lower the incidence of catheter-associated UTIs.

11. **Maintain a Healthy Diet:** A well-balanced diet that contains key nutrients is critical for seniors. Nutrient-rich diets may strengthen the immune system and general wellness.

12. **Avoid Irritants:** Encourage elders to avoid harsh soaps, scented products, and bubble baths that may irritate the genital region.

UTI Prevention During Pregnancy:

1. **Stay Hydrated:** Pregnant women should ensure they consume lots of water to preserve optimum hydration and urinary tract health. Increased fluid consumption may help wash out germs from the urinary system.

2. **Frequent Urination:** Respond swiftly to the desire to urinate. Holding in urine may raise the risk of UTIs, particularly during pregnancy when the uterus can exert pressure on the bladder.

3. **Cranberry Juice or Supplements:** Some pregnant women may consider drinking unsweetened cranberry juice or taking cranberry supplements to help prevent UTIs. Consult with a healthcare physician before beginning any new supplements.

4. **Urinate After Sexual Activity:** Ensure that you urinate after sexual activity to help flush out any germs that may have entered the urethra.

5. **Good Personal Hygiene:** Maintain good hygiene by keeping the genital region clean and dry.

6. **Avoid Irritants:** Refrain from using goods that may irritate the urinary system, such as bubble baths, harsh soaps, and scented products.

7. **Vaginal Health:** Discuss any concerns regarding vaginal health with your healthcare physician. They may advise on keeping a healthy vaginal environment.

8. **Quick Medical assistance:** If you develop signs of a UTI, such as discomfort during urination or frequent urine, get quick medical assistance, since untreated UTIs may lead to difficulties during pregnancy.

UTI Prevention for Individuals with Diabetes:

1. **Blood Sugar Control:** Proper control of blood sugar levels is necessary. Consistently high blood sugar levels may weaken the immune system and make the body more prone to infections, including UTIs.

2. **Stay Hydrated:** Adequate fluid consumption is vital for those with diabetes. It helps dilute urine and lower the incidence of UTIs.

3. **Regular Urination:** Respond immediately to the desire to urinate. Consistently elevated blood sugar levels might raise the risk of excessive urine.

4. **Excellent Hygiene:** Maintain excellent personal hygiene and keep the genital region clean and dry.

5. **Vaginal Health:** Discuss any concerns regarding vaginal health with your healthcare practitioner, since persons with diabetes may be more prone to vaginal yeast infections, which may raise the risk of UTIs.

6. **Frequent Medical Check-ups:** Attend frequent medical check-ups to monitor blood sugar management and general health.

UTI Prevention for Those with a History of Recurrent UTIs:

1. **Discuss with a Healthcare practitioner:** If you have a history of recurring UTIs, talk with your healthcare practitioner to determine any underlying reasons, contributing variables, or particular treatment techniques.

2. **Preventive Antibiotics:** In certain circumstances, a healthcare physician may prescribe low-dose antibiotics for long-term usage to prevent recurring UTIs.

3. **Tailored UTI Prevention Strategy: Work** with your healthcare physician to build a tailored UTI prevention strategy, which may include lifestyle changes, dietary adjustments, and specialized preventative measures.

4. **Regular Follow-up:** Continue to follow up with your healthcare physician for continuous monitoring and modifications to your UTI prevention strategy as required.

5. **Proper Personal Hygiene:** Maintain proper hygiene and avoid irritants that might provoke UTIs.

6. **Urgent Medical care:** If you develop symptoms of a UTI, get urgent medical care for early diagnosis and treatment.

Remember that individual situations might differ, and talking with a healthcare physician is crucial for specific UTI prevention techniques in these particular scenarios. UTI prevention may entail a mix of lifestyle modifications, medical treatments, and continued monitoring to lower the risk of recurring infections.

CHAPTER FOUR

DEALING WITH UTIs

Medicines to Treat UTIs

Urinary tract infections (UTIs) are commonly treated with antibiotics. The choice of antibiotic and the length of therapy rely on variables such as the kind of bacteria causing the illness and its sensitivity to antibiotics, the severity of the infection, and the patient's medical history. Here are some typical antibiotics used to treat UTIs:

1. **Trimethoprim/Sulfamethoxazole (TMP/SMX or Bactrim):** This combination antibiotic is effective against a broad spectrum of UTI-causing bacteria. It's typically used as a first-line therapy for uncomplicated UTIs.

2. **Nitrofurantoin (Macrodantin, Macrobid):** Nitrofurantoin is routinely used to treat UTIs and is appropriate for simple infections. It should be taken with food to improve absorption.

3. **Ciprofloxacin (Cipro) and Levofloxacin (Levaquin):**
   Fluoroquinolones like ciprofloxacin and levofloxacin are
   occasionally used to treat more severe or complex UTIs,
   particularly when the specific bacteria causing the infection
   are resistant to other antibiotics. They should be kept for
   circumstances where alternative solutions are not
   acceptable owing to probable negative effects.

4. **Cephalexin (Keflex) and Cefuroxime (Ceftin):** These
   cephalosporin antibiotics are occasionally administered for
   UTIs, especially when there is a known sensitivity to these
   medications.

5. **Amoxicillin/Clavulanate (Augmentin):** This combination
   antibiotic is used for more severe or complex UTIs and is
   occasionally recommended when there is suspicion of a
   larger range of bacteria causing the illness.

6. **Fosfomycin (Monurol):** Fosfomycin is a single-dose
   antibiotic typically used for uncomplicated UTIs. It may be
   effective in situations of known medication sensitivities or
   when choices are not suited.

7. Phenazopyridine (Pyridium): This drug is not an antibiotic but may give relief from the unpleasant symptoms of a UTI, such as burning during the urine. It should be used as a short-term symptomatic therapy and not as a replacement for antibiotics.

It's vital to follow the complete course of antibiotics as advised by your healthcare professional, even if you start feeling better before completing the medicine. This helps ensure full eradication of the illness and lowers the danger of antibiotic resistance.

If you develop severe or increasing symptoms, including fever, chills, back pain, or evidence of kidney involvement, get emergency medical assistance, as you may require intravenous (IV) antibiotics or hospitalization. Always follow your healthcare provider's instructions for treatment and communicate with them about any questions or concerns about your medicine.

Home Remedies for UTIs Relief

Here are some home treatments that might help ease UTI symptoms while you await medical treatment or alongside prescription antibiotics:

1. **Hydration:** Drink lots of water to help wash germs out of the urinary system. The objective is to maintain a healthy urine flow. Aim for at least 8-10 cups (64-80 ounces) of water every day.
2. **Cranberry Products:** Unsweetened cranberry juice or cranberry supplements may help prevent UTIs by making it tougher for germs to attach to the urinary system. While the data is conflicting, some individuals find these items useful.
3. **Frequent Urination:** Don't hold in urine for lengthy durations. Respond soon to the desire to urinate to flush away microorganisms.
4. **Warm Compress:** Applying a warm, moist heating pad or a warm water bottle to your lower belly will help ease pain and reduce pressure. Ensure it's not too hot to prevent burns.

5. **Over-the-counter pain medications:** Non-prescription pain medications like ibuprofen (Advil) or acetaminophen (Tylenol) may help decrease pain, discomfort, and fever. Follow suggested doses, and visit your healthcare practitioner if you have any concerns or are taking additional drugs.

6. **Probiotics:** Some research shows that probiotics containing helpful bacteria may help maintain a balanced flora in the urinary system. Discuss probiotic usage with your healthcare physician.

7. **Personal Hygiene:** Maintain proper personal hygiene, and use soft, unscented soap when washing the genital region to minimize irritation.

8. **Loose clothes:** Wear loose-fitting, breathable clothes to reduce irritation and enable sufficient ventilation.

9. **Avoid Sexual Activity:** While suffering UTI symptoms, it's suggested to avoid sexual activity to prevent additional discomfort and probable reinfection.

10. **Limit Caffeine and Alcohol**: Both caffeine and alcohol may function as diuretics, possibly contributing to

dehydration. If you want to drink these beverages, do so in moderation and ensure you keep appropriate hydration.

11. **Phenazopyridine (Pyridium):** This over-the-counter drug may give short relief from uncomfortable UTI symptoms, such as burning when urinating. It's a short-term symptomatic medication and not a replacement for antibiotics.

12. **Alternative therapy:** Some persons seek alternative therapy, such as D-mannose supplements, which may help prevent UTIs. Discuss these alternatives with your healthcare physician.

13. **Vitamin C:** Foods strong in vitamin C, such as citrus fruits and strawberries, may acidify the urine, perhaps making it difficult for germs to proliferate in the urinary system.

14. **Yogurt:** Consuming plain, unsweetened yogurt with live probiotic cultures may help maintain healthy gut and vaginal bacteria.

15.   **Avoid Irritants:** Steer away from harsh soaps, bubble baths, and fragrant feminine items that might increase symptoms.

16.   **Urinary Alkalinizers:** Some OTC urinary alkalinizers may help lessen UTI symptoms by making the urine less acidic. However, ask your healthcare physician before using them.

It's crucial to realize that although these home treatments might give relief from UTI symptoms, they do not address the underlying infection.

CHAPTER FIVE

RISKS AND LONG-TERM EFFECTS

Long-Term Effects

Urinary tract infections (UTIs) are frequent and, when properly recognized and treated, are typically not a reason for major worry. However, if left untreated or if they regularly return, UTIs may lead to severe consequences and health risks. Here are various complications that might emerge from UTIs:

1. **Kidney Infections (Pyelonephritis):** UTIs that extend to the kidneys may result in a more serious illness known as pyelonephritis. Symptoms may include high fever, chills, flank discomfort, and nausea. Kidney infections may be dangerous and need quick medical intervention.

2. **Repeated UTIs:** Some persons are prone to repeated UTIs, which may be uncomfortable and may suggest underlying concerns. Frequent antibiotic treatment to treat recurrent UTIs may lead to antibiotic resistance.

3. **Sepsis:** In extreme situations, a UTI may progress to sepsis, a life-threatening illness when the body's reaction to an infection produces extensive inflammation. Symptoms of sepsis include high temperature, fast heart rate, and disorientation. Sepsis demands prompt medical treatment.

4. **Kidney Damage**: Repeated or severe kidney infections may lead to kidney damage over time. This may affect kidney function and may need continuous medical care.

5. **Abscess development:** UTIs may lead to the development of abscesses in the kidneys, a collection of pus that may need surgical drainage or other procedures.

6. **Urethral Stricture:** In rare circumstances, persistent or recurring UTIs may lead to the narrowing of the urethra (urethral stricture), which can restrict the flow of urine.

7. **Bladder Infections (Cystitis):** While less serious than kidney infections, recurring or untreated UTIs may develop into chronic bladder infections (cystitis) that cause continuous discomfort and agony.

8. **Interstitial Cystitis:** In certain situations, repeated or chronic UTIs may progress to interstitial cystitis, a painful

illness characterized by persistent inflammation and irritation in the bladder.

9. **Pregnancy Complications:** UTIs during pregnancy might raise the risk of premature delivery and low birth weight. Proper care of UTIs is critical for pregnant women to reduce these risks.

10. **Complex UTIs:** Some UTIs might become complex owing to variables such as urinary tract anomalies, urinary blockage, or catheter usage. These may need a more prolonged course of antibiotics or extra therapies.

11. **Antibiotic Resistance:** Frequent or incorrect use of antibiotics to treat UTIs may develop into antibiotic resistance, where the bacteria become less susceptible to therapy. This makes subsequent infections more complex to control.

12. **Emotional and Quality of Life Impact:** Recurrent UTIs may lead to emotional anguish, worry, and a diminished quality of life owing to the pain and disturbance they create.

Living with UTIs That Don't Go Away

Living with persistent UTIs that don't go away, also known as chronic or recurrent UTIs, may be hard and disruptive to everyday life. However, there are techniques and lifestyle adjustments that may help manage your illness and enhance your quality of life. Here are some crucial elements to consider:

1. **Contact an expert:** If you're suffering from recurring or chronic UTIs, it's important to contact a urologist or infectious disease expert. These professionals have experience in addressing severe UTI situations and can give more tailored therapy choices.

2. **Uncover Underlying Causes:** Work with your healthcare practitioner to uncover any underlying issues contributing to your recurring UTIs. These may include anatomical defects, kidney stones, urine retention, diabetes, or other medical disorders. Addressing these underlying conditions may greatly lower the occurrence of infections.

3. **Preventive Antibiotics:** Your healthcare practitioner may suggest long-term, low-dose antibiotic treatment to prevent

recurring UTIs. This strategy, known as preventive or suppressive treatment, tries to lower the likelihood of subsequent infections. Follow your provider's advice and attend frequent check-ups to monitor your improvement.

4. **Behavioral and Lifestyle Changes:** Discuss with your healthcare practitioner any behavioral or lifestyle variables that may be contributing to your recurrent UTIs. This might involve sexual activity, hygienic behaviors, or food choices. Making suitable changes may help lower the risk of infection.

5. **Hormone Replacement Therapy (HRT):** If you're a postmenopausal woman and hormone changes are leading to UTIs, HRT may be prescribed. HRT may help restore hormonal balance and minimize sensitivity to UTIs. Consult with your healthcare practitioner for information on the most suited method.

6. **Vaginal Estrogen Cream:** Postmenopausal women may use vaginal estrogen cream to preserve the health of vaginal and urinary tract tissues, minimizing the incidence of UTIs.

7. **Probiotics:** Some persons get relief from recurring UTIs by utilizing probiotics containing helpful microorganisms. These may assist in maintaining a healthy balance of microorganisms in the urinary system. Consult with your healthcare practitioner to decide whether this is a viable choice for you.

8. **Hydration:** Proper hydration is necessary to preserve urinary tract health. Ensure you drink enough water to enable the regular flushing of germs from your urinary system. Aim for 8-10 cups (64-80 ounces) of water every day.

9. **Excellent Personal Hygiene:** Maintain excellent personal hygiene by using mild, unscented soap for cleansing the genital region and following adequate wiping methods.

10. **Stress Reduction:** High-stress levels might impair the immune system. Engage in stress-reduction practices such as meditation, yoga, deep breathing exercises, or therapy to support your general health and minimize the incidence of UTIs.

11. **Continual Follow-up:** Regularly follow up with your healthcare practitioner for continuous monitoring and modifications to your UTI prevention strategy. This enables your physician to analyze your progress and make any necessary modifications to your therapy.

Living with recurring UTIs may take tenacity and patience to identify the best effective treatment techniques. By engaging closely with your healthcare physician and investigating choices, you may better manage your condition and enhance your overall quality of life. If UTIs continue, consider these options with your healthcare physician to build a personalized strategy for your unique requirements.

CHAPTER SIX

THE FUTURE OF UTI CARE

New Ways to Treat UTIs

The treatment of urinary tract infections (UTIs) often requires antibiotics, which are efficient in eliminating the bacteria causing the illness. However, with increased concerns about antibiotic resistance and the need for more focused and less intrusive therapies, there is continuing research into novel and alternative approaches to treat UTIs. Here are some new and alternative approaches:

1. **Probiotics:** Probiotics, notably those containing beneficial bacteria like Lactobacillus species, have received attention for their potential to maintain a healthy balance of flora in the urinary system. By fighting with dangerous bacteria for resources and sticking to the urinary system, probiotics may help prevent UTIs. Research is continuing to find particular probiotic strains that are useful in preventing and treating UTIs.

2. **Vaccinations:** Developing vaccinations that target common UTI-causing bacteria is an attractive area of study. These vaccinations seek to boost the immune system to identify and kill germs more effectively, minimizing the risk of recurring UTIs. Vaccine development for UTIs is still at the experimental stage and needs additional research.

3. **Phage Therapy:** Bacteriophages, or "phages," are viruses that may infect and eliminate bacteria. Phage treatment is a promising subject where researchers are finding particular phages that may target and eliminate the bacteria responsible for UTIs. This technique provides the opportunity for individualized and highly focused therapy, which may be particularly advantageous in situations of antibiotic resistance.

4. **Antimicrobial Peptides:** Antimicrobial peptides are naturally occurring proteins that can damage bacterial cell walls and impede bacterial development. They are being examined for their potential in preventing and treating UTIs by directly targeting the bacteria responsible for the illness.

5. **Cranberry Products:** Cranberry juice or supplements have long been regarded as a natural cure for UTIs. The ongoing study is assessing the usefulness of cranberry products in preventing UTIs. It is suspected that some chemicals in cranberries may interfere with bacterial adherence to the urinary system walls.

6. **Local Antibiotics:** Some academics and healthcare practitioners are studying the use of localized antibiotic delivery. Antibiotics may be delivered directly into the urinary system by catheters or other means. This technique decreases systemic antibiotic exposure and may lessen the possibility of antibiotic resistance.

7. **Nanoparticles:** Nanoparticles loaded with antimicrobial drugs are being studied as a possible technique to administer targeted therapy to the urinary system. The use of nanoparticles may increase the effectiveness of therapy and lower the risk of negative effects associated with systemic antibiotics.

8. **Bladder Instillations:** Bladder instillations entail introducing medicine directly into the bladder via a

catheter. This approach offers targeted therapy for severe or recurring UTIs and may involve the use of drugs like dimethyl sulfoxide (DMSO) to reduce symptoms.

9. **Hyaluronic Acid Instillation:** Hyaluronic acid instillation is a treatment in which hyaluronic acid is infused into the bladder. It seeks to enhance the health of the bladder lining and lower the incidence of recurring UTIs.

10. **Electromagnetic Therapy:** Low-intensity electromagnetic fields are being explored for their potential in treating UTIs. They impede bacterial growth and biofilm development in the urinary system, which might make infections less severe and resistant to therapy.

11. **D-Mannose:** D-mannose is a sugar supplement that has gained appeal for its potential to prevent and control UTIs. It is supposed to interfere with bacterial attachment to the urinary system walls, avoiding infection.

12. **Chinese Herbal Medicine:** Traditional Chinese herbal medicine has been utilized for millennia in UTI treatment and prevention. Some herbal formulations are under research for their potential usefulness in controlling

UTIs. These formulations frequently comprise a mix of herbs that may offer antibacterial and anti-inflammatory effects.

While these developing medicines show promise, it's vital to underline that additional research and clinical studies are required to verify their safety and efficacy. Antibiotics remain the primary therapy for UTIs, particularly in severe or complex infections. As research progresses, these alternate techniques may provide significant choices for the management of UTIs. However, people should always contact a healthcare physician for the most suitable and evidence-based therapy for UTIs.

Exciting UTI Prevention Ideas

Preventing urinary tract infections (UTIs) is vital for maintaining excellent urological health. While certain preventative techniques are well-known, there are interesting and creative solutions that might help minimize the incidence of UTIs. Here are some inventive and interesting techniques for UTI prevention:

1. **Smart Hydration:** Hydration is vital in clearing away germs from the urinary system. Innovative hydration reminders and applications may help people measure their regular water consumption and urge them to keep appropriately hydrated.

2. **Wearable Technology:** Smart wearables, like fitness trackers and smart watches, can monitor hydration levels and remind users to drink water. They may also monitor toilet trips and assist in spotting any changes in urine patterns that may suggest an infection.

3. **Urine Health Apps:** There are growing mobile apps that concentrate on urine health. These applications may give vital information on UTI prevention, and hydration monitoring, and even link users with healthcare specialists for virtual consultations.

4. **Genetic Risk Assessment**: Genetic testing may identify people who are genetically prone to UTIs. Armed with this knowledge, individuals may take preventative steps targeted to their particular risk factors.

5. **Customised Probiotics:** Advancements in microbiome research have brought up the prospect of customized probiotics tailored to an individual's specific microbial makeup. These probiotics may establish a healthy balance of urinary tract bacteria and lower the risk of infection.

6. **Vaginal microbiota Health:** Some UTIs are connected to abnormalities in the vaginal microbiota. Innovative therapies concentrate on repairing and maintaining a healthy vaginal flora to lower UTI risk.

7. **Biocompatible Materials:** Researchers are studying the development of biocompatible materials for urinary catheters and other medical devices to lower the likelihood of bacterial adhesion and biofilm formation, ultimately decreasing catheter-associated UTIs.

8. **Nano-Coatings:** Nano-coatings on catheters, urine bags, and other medical equipment may make these devices more resistant to bacterial adherence, lessening the risk of infections in healthcare settings.

9. **Behavioral Intervention Apps:** Apps intended to improve habits that raise UTI risks, such as poor cleanliness or

insufficient water, may give users real-time guidance and assistance.

10. **Telemedicine Consultations:** Telemedicine and virtual healthcare platforms enable users to consult with healthcare professionals rapidly, making it simpler to address UTIs and obtain prompt treatment.

11. **Cranberry-Delivery methods:** Novel delivery methods for cranberry chemicals, which are expected to impede bacterial adherence to urinary tract walls, may give more convenient and effective choices for UTI prevention.

12. **Urine Testing Kits:** Home urine testing kits are becoming more available and may help people check their urinary health frequently, identify early indications of illness, and seek medical care when required.

13. **Behavioral therapy:** Behavioral therapy and support, either in-person or via telehealth services, may assist patients with reoccurring UTIs in achieving permanent changes in hygiene habits and lifestyle choices that minimize their risk.

14. **Community Education:** Innovative community-based health initiatives may promote awareness about UTI prevention and offer resources and assistance to high-risk communities.

15. **Biometric Devices:** Advances in biometric technology enable non-invasive monitoring of urine parameters. These gadgets may assist in identifying early indicators of urinary tract malfunction and allow appropriate therapies.

16. **Artificial Intelligence:** AI-powered healthcare solutions may evaluate data from wearables, mobile applications, and biometric devices to deliver individualized suggestions for UTI prevention.

CONCLUSION

In conclusion, urinary tract infections (UTIs) are frequent, although generally underestimated, health issues that impact millions of persons globally. While often seen as straightforward and manageable, UTIs may have far-reaching ramifications for one's well-being.

This book has studied every part of UTIs, from their origins and symptoms to prevention and treatment, and even the developing, creative ways for treating and avoiding these infections. We've dug into the possible problems and long-term implications of UTIs, underlining the significance of early identification and adequate therapy.

Moreover, we've stressed the significance of UTI prevention, including lifestyle modifications, cleanliness habits, and preventive measures, as the cornerstone of urinary health. We've also studied the dynamic world of research and innovation, revealing fresh insights and fascinating breakthroughs that may define the future of UTI prevention and care.

Ultimately, the information learned from this book provides you with the skills to not only diagnose and manage UTIs but also to assume a proactive role in your urinary health. It underlines the value of cooperation with healthcare professionals, as well as the potential of research and innovation in transforming the landscape of UTI prevention and treatment.

As you continue on your road towards keeping a healthy urinary tract and general well-being, remember that information is your greatest advantage. be educated, be proactive, and, most importantly, stay healthy. Your urinary health is a vital component of your overall health, and it's worth every effort to safeguard and respect it.